Problems with Meat

Problems with Meat

John A. Scharffenberg, M.D., M.P.H.

Associate Professor of Applied Nutrition
Loma Linda University
Director, Community Health Education
San Joaquin Community Hospital
Bakersfield, California

Based on a presentation at an annual meeting of the
American Association for the Advancement of Science
Washington, D.C.

Published by
Woodbridge Press Publishing Company
Santa Barbara, California 93111

Second printing 1982

Published by

Woodbridge Press Publishing Company
Post Office Box 6189
Santa Barbara, California 93111

Published simultaneously in the United States and Canada

Printed in the United States of America

Library of Congress Cataloging in Publication Data

Scharffenberg, John A
  Problems with meat.

  "Based on a presentation at an annual meeting of the American
Association for the Advancement of Science, Washington, D.C."

  Includes bibliographical references.
  1. Meat.   2. Nutritionally induced diseases.
I. American Association for the Advancement of
Science.   II. Title. [DNLM: 1. Meat—Adverse
effects.   2. Vegetarianism.   WB426 S311p]
TX556.M4S34   613.2′8   79-13056
ISBN 0-912800-65-8

Contents

List of Tables and Figures

7

Preface

If meat, as a human food source, had only one problem to be discussed it could easily be fully accomplished in the space of this book. There are so many problems, however, that what I shall do here is briefly describe them, provide enough scientific data to establish the reality and seriousness of the problems, and provide a framework of discussion that will enable interested persons to pursue in detail the areas of greatest personal interest.

I will also suggest practical steps for improvements in diet and life-style that will help readers to reduce their chances of contracting the "killer" diseases so prevalent in our society and to increase the possibility of a longer and healthier life.

John A. Scharffenberg, M.D.

Meat–Dangerous and Difficult

It may startle you to know that next to tobacco and alcohol, the use of meat is probably the greatest single cause of mortality in the United States. This is likely also the case in some other "affluent" societies.

It may also startle you to know that, contrary to common opinion, it is *more difficult* to have a good diet *with* meat than without it—and that you don't have to worry about complicated "protein supplementation" to have ample proteins, in both quality and quantity, in a simple vegetarian diet.

Problems with Meat

First, a word about the dangers of meat. Scientific curiosity about—and consequently, scientific study of—the effects of meat on health and longevity is now beginning to catch up with similar work that has long since established the tragic effects of alcohol and tobacco on the human system. The knowledge these scientific inquiries have already produced about the harmful effects of meat, and what you can do with this knowledge to improve and extend your own life is what this book is about.

Studies conducted over the past few years have established to the satisfaction of a large number of medical and scientific professionals that meat is an undesirable food for at least these six reasons:

1. Meat is a major contributor to the leading causes of death.

2. The cost of meat is excessively high in relation to nutritional value.

3. The production of meat as food wastes energy and other resources.

4. Meat is deficient in two major food components: fiber and carbohydrates.

5. Contrary to popular belief, it is actually difficult to achieve good nutrition utilizing a flesh diet.

6. The best alternative diet, not based on meat, has none of these problems.

In this book I will tell you enough about the alternatives to meat to give you a solid grasp of life-supporting nutritional patterns. I will also give you the evidence that with a vegetarian diet you don't have to have a "complete" protein at every meal or even necessarily each day.

In fact, if you are maintaining your ideal body weight it is almost impossible to be protein deficient.

But first, let's look at the striking evidence that one of man's oldest dietary habits, the use of meat as food, is—quite literally—killing him.

Potential Health Hazards in the Use of Meat

Problems with the use of meat as a human food source may be discussed from three major standpoints:

1. Potential disease hazards in the use of meat
2. The population explosion and economics
3. Nutritional problems with meat

First, current scientific evidence about the disease potential—the relation of meat to these specific major problems—will be presented:

1. Atherosclerosis
2. Cancer
3. Decrease in longevity or life expectancy
4. Kidney disorders
5. Salmonellosis
6. Osteoporosis
7. Trichinosis

Meat and Atherosclerosis

For a long time there has been a general belief that a meat-based diet is somehow related to atherosclerosis, a thickening of the walls of arteries associated with heart attacks, strokes, and other problems. As early as 1961, editorials in the *Journal of the American Medical Association* made statements like this: "A vegetarian diet can prevent 97 percent of our coronary occlusions "(23)

Since that time the risk factors for atherosclerosis and heart disease have become scientifically well identified, in large part through several well-organized studies.

Problems with Meat

Inter-Society Commission for Heart Disease Resources

Twenty-nine voluntary health agencies, including the American Medical Association, formed a joint commission to identify the risk factors of atherosclerosis and heart attacks and to tell the American public what to do to stem this "epidemic." The Inter-Society Commission appointed two study groups consisting of many of the nation's top scientists. In 1970, they reported these findings:

Major risk factors of atherosclerosis and heart attacks are:

1. High blood lipids (fat molecules, mainly cholesterol and triglycerides)
2. High blood pressure
3. Cigarette smoking

Recommendations were then made regarding diet for the control of blood lipids. They included:

1. Correction of obesity
2. Reduction of dietary cholesterol to 300 mg. per day
3. Reduction of dietary saturated fat to less than 10 percent of the total calories
4. Reduction of total fat to less than 35 percent of calorie intake.

Recommendations included:

1. Avoiding egg yolks, bacon, lard and suet
2. Greater use of grains, fruits, vegetables and legumes.

"It is necessary," they stated, "to encourage further development of high quality vegetable protein products." (42)

Senate Select Committee on Nutrition and Human Needs

In 1977, the Senate Select Committee on Nutrition and Human Needs, after extended study of the health effects of various dietary patterns, adopted and published a remarkable document: *United States Dietary Goals*. (78) These goals include:

1. Increase of carbohydrate consumption to 55–60 percent of calories
2. Decrease in total fat from 40 to 30 percent of calories
3. Decrease in saturated fat to 10 percent of calories
4. Decrease in cholesterol to 300 mg. per day
5. Decrease in sugar by 40 percent to 15 percent of calories
6. Decrease in salt by 50–85 percent to 3 gm. per day (later liberalized to 5 gm. per day)

Attaining these goals, the committee suggests the following changes in dietary habits:

1. Increase in use of fruits, vegetables and whole grains
2. Decrease in use of red meat and increase in use of poultry and fish
3. Decrease in use of high-fat foods

Problems with Meat

4. Use of nonfat milk
5. Decrease in use of butterfat, eggs, and other high-cholesterol foods
6. Decrease in use of sugar and foods high in sugar
7. Decrease in use of salt and foods high in salt.

This is the most outstanding nutritional statement ever produced by political leaders in the United States. It has won applause from many health and nutritional scientists.

It is clear that, at the very top, scientific and political groups alike have come to the conclusion that the American diet should be improved—and that the principal recommendations center on the use of less red meat and associated products.

There have been numerous scientific studies that support these recommendations. Let's look at just a few of them.

Finnish Mental Hospital Study

Men in two mental hospitals in Finland were compared. In one hospital, whole milk was replaced by milk that contained soybean oil instead of butterfat, and butter was replaced by soft margarine—thus decreasing saturated fat in the diet. The second hospital was used as a control with no changes. In neither hospital was there any change in the meat in the diet because the researchers did not want the men to be aware that a study was being conducted. Yet the study was based on the theory that saturated fats elevate serum cholesterol, which in turn increases the risk of heart attacks.

The experimental hospital patients stayed on their special diet for six years, during which their serum cholesterol was greatly reduced. They were then returned to the "normal" diet and their serum cholesterol rose again. At the beginning of a second six-year period, the original "control" hospital changed from the "normal" to the experimental special diet with the same results—lowered serum cholesterol levels for the patients.

The serum cholesterol of patients in the experimental hospital was reduced from an average of 266 to 217 mg/100 ml. and the death rates based on per-1,000-person-years from coronary heart disease was reduced from 13.0 to 5.7. Patients' serum cholesterol in the other hospital was reduced from 268 to 234 mg./100 ml. and death rates from 15.2 to 7.5.

Thus, a reduction of more than one-half of the coronary heart disease mortality was achieved by changing only two items in the diet! The investigators also concluded that total mortality rates among the patients was also favorably affected by the altered diet. (56)

Problems with Meat

Seventh-day Adventists and Coronary Heart Disease

Because the use of meat is discouraged and smoking is forbidden among members of the Seventh-day Adventist church, and because of other special characteristics of their life-style, that group continues to be studied by health scientists. Some of the findings are striking.

For example, Seventh-day Adventist men aged 35–40 have a 6.2 years' greater life expectancy than men in the general population. (47) When compared with non-smokers only, the life expectancy advantage is still 3.1 years. (47) Thus, one-half of their advantage is due to the fact that they do not smoke. The other half is due to some other factor or factors. Even if in the general population all cancer deaths (the second leading cause of mortality) were avoided, the increase in life expectancy would still not bring the life expectancy up to that seen among the Seventh-day Adventist group. Therefore, the factor giving this group the greater advantage must be related primarily to the greatest cause of mortality, atherosclerosis and its associated problems.

Seventh-day Adventist men have only 54 percent of the expected mortality from coronary heart disease. (67) Adventists do have heart attacks but they occur approximately 10 years later in life. The common denominator in this lowered mortality from heart disease is a diet that contains much less meat.

A recent study comparing Adventists who had differing dietary habits showed observed-to-expected coronary heart disease mortality as follows: (67)

Observed-to-Expected Coronary Heart Disease Mortality

Adventist Men

Meat Users	64%
Lacto-Ovo-Vegetarians	40%
Total Vegetarians	23%

Problems with Meat

Again, this illustrates that saturated fats tend to increase heart disease. Meat users among the Adventist group do not smoke and probably use less meat than men in the general population, accounting for their lowered mortality rate. Lacto-ovo-vegetarian Adventist men (using dairy products and eggs) have still lower coronary heart disease mortality rates. Total vegetarians have rates approximately one-third that of meat users.

An even more recent study from this group shows that total vegetarian Adventist men have only 12 percent of the expected coronary heart disease mortality, based on that occurring in the general population.(68)

This is one of the most revealing studies of the past decade. It points out that not only can heart disease mortality be reduced but that life expectancy can be increased. It also establishes beyond reasonable doubt that saturated fat, and specifically meat, is a factor in heart disease mortality. This study does not compare peoples of different cultures or groups with many variables but compares groups with variables held relatively constant except for the dietary factors of meat, milk, and eggs.

Atherosclerosis begins early in life. We recently conducted a study in Bakersfield, California, of age-sex-height-weight-matched high school children at the Garces Catholic High School and the Adventist Academy. This study demonstrated the differences in dietary habits and the corresponding differences in serum lipids, cholesterol, and triglycerides, all major factors in atherosclerosis. (See tables—one presenting the highlights, the other presenting more detail.)

Diet Lipid Study

(Bakersfield, California, Parochial School Students)

	ADVENTIST *(Low Meat Use)*		CATHOLIC *(Normal Meat Use)*	
	Male	*Female*	*Male*	*Female*
Serum Cholesterol, mg. %	162	162	188	214
% Students Above 180 mg. Serum Cholesterol	21	23	61	88
Serum Triglycerides, mg. %	63	63	73	75
%Students Who Ate Beef Three or More Times Per Week	21	24	86	69

Diet-Lipid Study Results
Adventist Students and Catholic Students
(28 Boys, 26 Girls—Age-Sex-Height-Weight-Matched)

	Adventist Students (low meat use)		Catholic Students (normal meat use)	
	Boys	*Girls*	*Boys*	*Girls*
Serum Cholesterol, mg% (mean)	162	162	188	214
Serum Cholesterol, mg% (median)	152-3	155-160	188	210-214
% Students Above 180 mg%	21%	23%	61%	88%
Serum Cholesterol, mg% range	111-291	105-245	136-239	169-274
Serum Triglycerides, mg% (mean)	63	63	73	75
Serum Triglycerides, mg% (median)	59-61	60-61	69-70	70-72
Serum Triglycerides, mg% range	30-129	30-105	34-144	35-129
%Students Lacto-Ovo Vegetarians	29%	46%	0%	0%
No. Students Smoking	0	0	1	0
%Using Bacon 3× or More/Week	0%	0%	32%	12%
% Using Beef 3× or More/Week	21%	24%	86%	69%
% Using Cheese 3× or More/Week	32%	44%	46%	42%
% Using Ice Cream 3× or More/Week	14%	12%	57%	23%
% Using 4 or More Eggs/Week	11%	38%	32%	42%
% Using Candy 4× or More/Week	11%	12%	46%	35%
% Using 5 or More Colas/Week	21%	15%	50%	19%
% Using 3 or More Cups Whole Milk/Day	18%	31%	21%	38%
% For which a Cardiorespiratory Type of Physical Fitness Program Was Recommended	32%	35%	14%	19%

Studies of persons in later life, as stated, predictably show Adventist men who possibly have had lower levels of serum lipids since childhood, to have only 54 percent of the expected coronary heart disease mortality.(67)

Many other studies also show that diet can reduce heart disease. The reader may wish to look up some of them, such as the Los Angeles Veteran's Administration Hospital study (20) and the Anti-Coronary Club study of New York City.(15)

Norwegian Study

Comparison of death rates from circulatory diseases in Norway during pre– and post–World War II years versus the war years themselves—when animal fats were scarce—again supports the saturated fat–heart-disease theory. (84) The accompanying graph shows strikingly how the "deprivation" of animal fats during the war resulted in a remarkably lower death rate.

You may wish to study the full report by Malmros, which presents well the dietary changes in various Scandinavian countries during the war and the corresponding low mortality rates.(51)

The Prudent Diet

Scientists (42) and political groups (78) are recommending anew the Prudent Diet for the prevention of heart disease. This is the diet that Dr. Norman Jolliffe of New York City's Bureau of Nutrition used some time ago in an "anti-coronary club"—a diet that reduced the incidence of heart problems by one-half during a ten-year period.

Problems with Meat

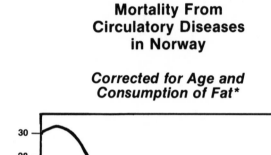

**Mortality From
Circulatory Diseases
in Norway**

*Corrected for Age and
Consumption of Fat**

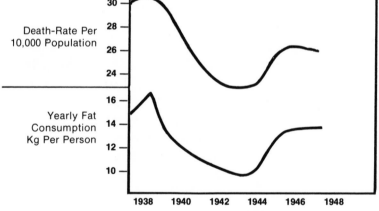

*In form of butter, milk, cheese and eggs.

28

The Prudent Diet is low in fat, meat, cholesterol, saturated fat, and calories, and high in fruits, whole grains, vegetables, and legumes.

The American Health Foundation supports the Prudent Diet. Dr. Ernst Wynder states:

> We and others have recommended a so-called "Prudent Diet" as a preventive approach to atherogenic disease.
>
> We suggest that a similar diet . . . be followed as a possible means of reducing the incidence of certain cancers.(90)

Dr. Mark Hegsted, formerly of Harvard University also supports the dietary changes implicit in the Prudent Diet. He states:

> Americans eat too much food. They eat too much meat, too much fat—especially saturated fat—too much cholesterol, too much salt, too much sugar. They should cut their consumption of these and increase their consumption of fruits, vegetables and cereal products—especially whole grains.(37)

A Summary: Atherosclerosis/Heart Disease

It is now known that serum cholesterol and thus atherosclerosis can be reduced by proper diet. Morbidity and mortality rates from coronary heart disease also can be lowered by dietary means. Total mortality rates (from all causes combined) may be reduced through diet, and thus life expectancy may be increased.

Problems with Meat

Reversal of the pathologic changes of atherosclerosis can be accomplished in monkeys through a diet based on the saturated fat theory, but such reversal cannot yet be said to have definitely occurred in current studies of human beings. But the argument should not be, "Can one reverse atherosclerosis?" when it is well known that heart disease mortality, mostly due to atherosclerosis, can be reduced and life expectancy increased by a change in diet and other habits of life.

The Prudent Diet, one which is low in fat, meat, and cholesterol, and high in fruits, whole grains, vegetables, and legumes, conforms to the best scientific information available and to the United States dietary goals as established by the Senate Select Committee on Nutrition and Human Needs.

Meat and Cancer

Meat is implicated in a wide variety of factors and processes known to be associated with a potential for cancer. These include the following—and in each case some remarkable information is available that will cause you to think seriously about whether you really want to include meat in your diet:

1. Chemical carcinogens
2. Cancer virus
3. Lessened host resistance
4. Lack of fiber
5. Rapid maturation
6. High-fat diet
7. High prolactin levels

Problems with Meat

Chemical Carcinogens

In 1 kg. (2.2 lbs.) of charcoal-broiled steak there is as much benzopyrene as in the smoke from 600 cigarettes.(49) When mice are fed benzopyrene they develop stomach tumors and leukemia.(72)

When the fat of meat is superheated, methylcholanthrene, a carcinogenic substance, is formed. When given to mice in subcarcinogenic doses, it makes them more susceptible to cancer from other carcinogens also given at subcarcinogenic levels.(64) Small doses increase cancer susceptibility.

Seventy percent of pork products have added nitrites to protect against botulism-like organisms and to promote "fresh" color. Nitrites combined with secondary and tertiary amines may produce nitrosamines, which are carcinogenic agents.(17) And one cannot avoid those "secondary and tertiary amines" because they are found in innumerable foods in the natural state. The government is limiting the amount of nitrites used in pork and other animal products.

Cancer Virus

Cancer viruses are found in tumors in animals. It was demonstrated long ago that these viruses can be transmitted from one animal to another within the same species. Peyton Rous in 1910 was able to demonstrate this transfer with chicken sarcomas. Bittner in the 1930s was able to induce mammary tumors in young mice nursed by mothers with breast tumors. The cancer virus was evidently transmitted through the milk.

Benzopyrene
(Carcinogen Related to Stomach Tumors and Leukemia)

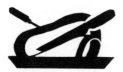 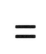

The amount from
1 kg. charcoal broiled steak

The amount from
600 cigarettes

Problems with Meat

It has now been demonstrated that cancer viruses can also be transmitted from an animal of one species to an animal of another species. Human leukemic tissue injected into small animals produced no leukemia but did produce other types of cancer—cancer of the breast, lungs, etc. (32, 33)

In 1974 it was shown that chimpanzees fed since birth with milk from leukemic cows died of leukemia in the first year of life.(83) After reporting this study, the American Cancer Society's journal, *CA–A Cancer Journal for Clinicians*, states simply, "Comment to stimulate a sense of urgency appears superfluous."

It is, of course, unethical to attempt to produce cancer in human beings. Therefore, actual proof that humans get cancer from animals is still lacking. However, "It is hardly possible for a virologist to think that family relatives of the numerous tumor viruses of animals will find no expression in the human species."(40)

Lessened Host Resistance

Diets with beef tallow (unlike corn oil) affect cell walls in insects, producing a more open and perhaps vulnerable latticework-like membrane. The possibility that this effect increases susceptibility to invasive disease needs to be studied.(7) Dietary factors have been shown to affect host resistance.

Lack of Fiber

Colon cancer is the predominant type of cancer in the United States and the second leading cause of cancer

Progressive Evidence of
Virus Transmission Between
Animals and Man

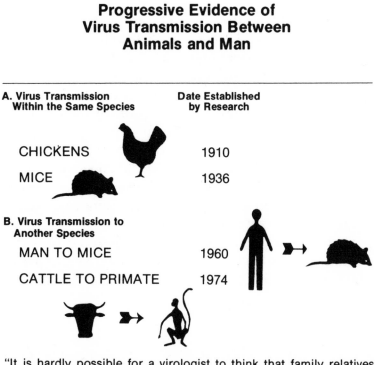

**A. Virus Transmission
Within the Same Species**

**Date Established
by Research**

CHICKENS 1910

MICE 1936

**B. Virus Transmission to
Another Species**

MAN TO MICE 1960

CATTLE TO PRIMATE 1974

"It is hardly possible for a virologist to think that family relatives of the numerous tumor viruses of animals will find no expression in the human species."

— *Public Health Report
January, 1959, p. 12*

35

Problems with Meat

mortality. Colon cancer occurs in the United States 8–15 times more frequently than in countries where the populace lives on a largely unrefined diet with greater fiber content.(19)

A relevant fact is that the average transit time through the gastrointestinal tract on an unrefined diet is 30 hours, versus 77 hours on a refined diet.(11)

It is also interesting that persons in countries where there is a high colon cancer rate tend to produce more bile acids than persons living in countries where colon cancers are rare—and that colon cancer patients also produce more bile acids.(90) A study has shown that two bile acids, lithocholic and taurodeoxycholic, enhanced cancer growth when applied to large bowel of rats.(90) Adequate fiber in the diet may help to remove these bile acids from the gastrointestinal tract.

Certain types of fiber such as those found in oats, (21) pectin, (44) and legumes (54) also help to lower serum cholesterol, which results in less potential for coronary heart disease.

In view of these facts it is quite alarming that so much of the diet of the average American consists of foods with low fiber content. Note in this table that meat is one of the main sources of food that provides little fiber:

Percentage of Calories from Foods with Little Fiber

Meat	20%
Refined Cereals	18%
Visible Fats	18%
Sugar	17%
Milk	12%
Eggs	2%
Alcohol	2%
Total	89%

Low Fiber Foods Predominate in Modern Refined Diet

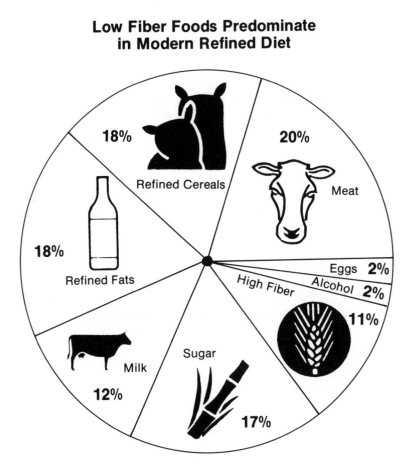

18%
Refined Cereals

20%
Meat

18%
Refined Fats

Eggs 2%
Alcohol 2%
High Fiber
11%

12%
Milk

Sugar
17%

Low Fiber Foods 89%

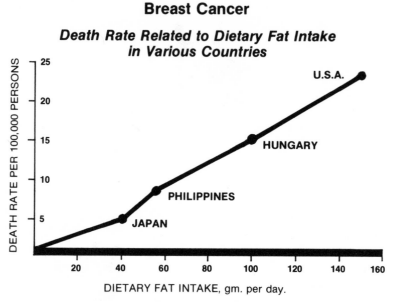

Breast Cancer

*Death Rate Related to Dietary Fat Intake
in Various Countries*

Adapted from K.K. Carroll

Rapid Maturation

Studies by T. Hirayama of the National Cancer Center Research Institute of Japan show that girls with early menarche (onset of menstrual period), under 13 years of age, compared with those with menarche over 17 years of age have 4.2 times greater incidence of breast cancer. (39)

Rapid maturation occurs in animals on high-protein diets. Vegetarians mature more slowly, as evidenced by permanent teeth coming in later in life, "growth spurt" coming later, and a delay in menarche. (45)

High-Fat Diet

It has been suggesed that it is the high fat content of a diet based on meat that is the principle cause of breast cancer. In countries with higher fat consumption breast cancer mortality rates increase. (14) This rate correlates with total fat, with animal fat, and with animal protein—but not with vegetable fat. (13) In this table Hirayama shows the risk of breast cancer in Japan relative to the use of meat, eggs, butter and cheese: (39)

Relative Risk of Breast Cancer

	Meat	Eggs	Butter/Cheese
Less than 1x/Week	1.00	1.00	1.00
2-4x/Week	2.55	1.91	3.23
Almost Daily	3.83	2.86	2.10

Problems with Meat

Breast Cancer

Correlation With Frequency of Meat in the Diet

MEAT SERVINGS PER WEEK	RELATIVE RISK
<1	1.00
2-4	2.55
7 or more	3.83

Breast Cancer
Correlation with Certain Dietary Patterns

FREQUENCY OF USE		EGGS	BUTTER, CHEESE
About once per week		1.00	1.00
2 - 4 times per week		1.91	3.23
Daily		2.86	2.10

Problems with Meat

Note that the risk of breast cancer increases most strikingly among users of meat, in proportion to the amount used. In Japan, pork is commonly used because beef is so costly. Breast cancer correlated most closely with pork usage.

Other studies have noted that among those using a high-fat diet there are not only more breast cancers but also more colon and prostate cancers.(90)

Still other studies showed that Americans consuming a mixed Western diet (high in meat) have four to five times more production of bile acids than do Seventh-day Adventist vegetarians and other American vegetarians, as well as Japanese and Chinese. (71) Since it has been shown that certain bile acids enhance colon tumor formation, such studies appear to be significant.(71)

High Prolactin Levels

A high-fat diet tends to increase the nighttime surge of prolactin, (90) a pituitary hormone promoting milk formation and lactation. The prolactin-estrogen ratio is thereby increased. High prolactin levels enhance mammary tumor growth in animals. When humans change from a meat diet to a vegetarian diet, the prolactin surge appears to be reduced to almost one-half that noted while on a meat diet. (90) A Western-type diet tends to increase the incidence of breast cancer. This diet is high in fat, meat, milk, and cholesterol.

Production of Bile Acids
in Vegetarians

	American Population in General	Seventh-Day Adventists, Other Vegetarians, Japan, China, U.S.A.
	mg/day	
Total Bile Acids	260	50
Deoxycholic Acids	110	30
Lithocholic Acids	85	20

Problems with Meat

Seventh-day Adventists and Cancer

**Mortality From Cancers
Not Related to Smoking
and Drinking:**   50-70% of that of
                         General Population

Adventist Diet: 25% Less Fat
                         50% More Fiber

Adventist Colon Cancer:
Relative Risk
                   Never Used Meat   **1.0**
                   Used Meat in the Past   **2.8**
                   Present Use of Beef   **2.3**
                   Present Use of Lamb   **2.7**

Seventh-day Adventists and Cancer

Among Seventh-day Adventists, the mortality from cancers not related to smoking and drinking is only 50–70 percent as great as that in the general population. (66) The Adventist diet consists of 25 percent less fat and 50 percent more fiber than that of the general population. (66) About half of the group uses no meat and the remainder may use some, but usually less than persons in the general population.

Breast cancer among women graduating from the University of Southern California medical school is much greater than among women graduating from Loma Linda University medical school, an Adventist institution. (65)

Breast cancer among Seventh-day Adventists shows a great deal of difference in rates among Adventist vegetarians compared with Adventist nonvegetarians. Vegetarians had the lowest mortality rates (only 65 percent of the expected death rate); those who ate meat three times a week or less had a higher rate (85 percent of the expected death rate); while those who used it more than three times a week had the highest rate (118 percent of the expected death rate). (69) A dose-response relationship is one of the tests used to demonstrate a cause-and-effect relationship. Obese women in this group have breast cancer mortality rates similar to those found in the general population, but those who are normal in weight have much lower rates. (69)

A small case study of the risk of colon cancer for Adventists relative to their differing dietary habits showed the following:

Problems with Meat

Adventist Colon Cancer: Relative Risk

Non-Meat Users   1.0
Present Beef Users   2.3
Present Lamb Users   2.7

The author summarizes, "This strongly suggests that the lacto-ovo-vegetarian diet may protect against colon cancer."(66) Larger studies do not show this great a difference based on varying dietary patterns. However, Adventists in general do have only 72 percent of the expected incidence of colon cancer. Perhaps a combination of less fat and more fiber are the decisive factors.

Breast Cancer

Women Medical Graduates

UNIVERSITY OF SOUTHERN CALIFORNIA (Normal Meat Use)	LOMA LINDA UNIVERSITY (Low Meat Use)

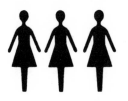

Problems with Meat

Breast Cancer Mortality
of Seventh Day Adventists
As Compared to the General Population

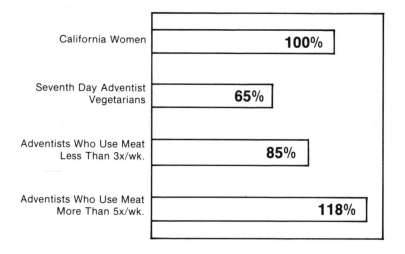

California Women — 100%

Seventh Day Adventist Vegetarians — 65%

Adventists Who Use Meat Less Than 3x/wk. — 85%

Adventists Who Use Meat More Than 5x/wk. — 118%

Longevity

In the light of scientific evidence, the ancient scriptural attribution of a shortened life span to meat eating seems dramatically pertinent. According to the biblical record the average age of the first ten patriarchs from Adam to Noah was 912 years. After this time meat became a part of the diet of man and the record states (Genesis 9:3–5) that one result would be a shorter life span. Thus, the next ten generations recorded, between Shem and Abraham, lived an average of only 317 years. (Even though meat was permitted, the fat of the animal was not supposed to be eaten [Lev. 3:17]. The same rule applied to Christians of the New Testament [Acts 15:20].)

Animal studies tend to support this biblical record. A high-protein diet throughout the life span shortens life

Problems with Meat

expectancy in rats. Rapid growth and short life go together. (80, 81, 46, 75, 26) Ross demonstrated that of the 17–23 enzymes studied in small animals, most were at the levels found in young animals when on a low-protein diet—but the levels found commonly in old animals when on a high-protein diet. (74, 76) Meat is a high-protein food and when used in large quantities appears to not be conducive to long life.

Effect of High Protein Diet on Life Expectancy

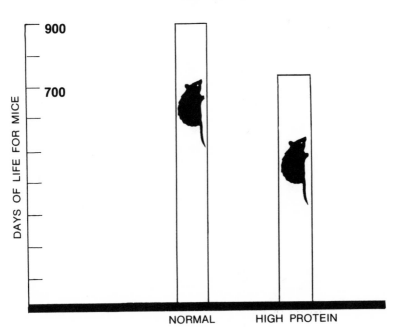

Kidney Disorders

It has long been known that a high-protein diet tends to cause kidney enlargement and nephritis (inflammation of the kidneys) in rats. (25) This results when protein accounts for more than 20 percent of the calories in their diet. Many Americans get that much protein in their diet.

More recently a study of cows demonstrated hypertrophy, or enlargement, of the kidneys from a high-protein diet. (82) Veterinarians noted more kidney disease in animals after pet foods containing 100 percent meat were placed on the market.

The body must rid itself of excess protein. It steps up the protein turnover rate, the protein half-life is shortened, the proteins are more rapidly degraded, and the additional nitrogen is processed in the liver and excreted in the urine. This means more work for the liver and kidneys, and these organs gradually hypertrophy or enlarge to take care of the load. (82)

Salmonellosis

Salmonellosis is a bacterial infection derived from contaminated animal food products. There are an estimated 2,000,000 cases of salmonellosis annually. The yearly cost is estimated at $300,000,000. It is usually only a miserable nuisance except for the aged, the ill, and infants, who may die from this disease. Death is estimated to result in 0.22 percent of the cases.

The problem is increasing and as long as people use meat as food the salmonellosis problem is not likely to be conquered. The National Academy of Science reports, "Reluctantly, we are forced to recognize the infeasibility of eradicating salmonellosis at this time." (61)

Osteoporosis

The Food and Nutrition Board of the National Research Council has for many years recommended an allowance of calcium in the American diet at the extremely high level of 800 mg. per day. (28) But in many countries a 300 to 400 mg. per day intake is common with no more osteoporosis or other calcium deficiency problems than are noted in this country. The Interdepartmental Committee on Nutrition for National Defense recommended only 400 mg. per day in the developing countries where they conducted nutritional surveys. (41)

Why is a very high level of calcium intake recommended for the United States population and only half that amount for persons in developing countries? The answer lies in the amount of protein used and the important calcium-to-phosphorus ratio in the diet. In 1960, the ratio in the American diet was 1 to 2.8 but now is approaching 1 to 4 due to less use of milk, more use of

Problems with Meat

meat, and more soft drinks, which contain phosphoric acid. (50) Skull osteoporosis occurs in monkeys fed a diet of table scraps with a calcium-to-phosphorous ratio of 1 to 5. (50)

A very high calcium intake is necessary in the United States diet because a high-protein diet increases the urinary excretion of calcium. In one study, men 18–20 years of age were given protein ranging from 48–141 gm. daily. The higher levels of protein doubled the urinary excretion of calcium when both the calcium and phosphorus intake were held constant at 1400 mg. (43) Other studies corroborate these findings. (52, 2)

A diet high in meat with its high protein content will therefore increase the urinary excretion of calcium. "It has been established that the extracellular fluid calcium levels are maintained at the expense of bone calcium and that a negative balance over a long period of time results in diminution of bone mass and osteoporosis." (2)

Bone responds to an acid ash load by dissolution of its basic salts. The loss of only 2 milliequivalents of calcium per day would in ten years account for a 15 percent loss of inorganic bone mass. (88) Vegetarians have significantly greater bone densities than omnivores; (24) thus vegetarians appear to be less prone to osteoporosis. (24)

In fact, it has just recently been shown that bone calcium is at dangerously low levels (where fractures could easily occur) in those using meat as compared to vegetarians, especially in the over-50-year age group. This was discovered in a study of 1,000 persons age-sex matched between vegetarians and nonvegetarians. (53).

Trichinosis

In some countries trichinosis is reason enough for avoiding the use of meat. In the United States, fortunately, trichinosis is becoming less common. The National Center for Disease Control reports:

A recent autopsy study has shown that 4.3 percent of 5,000 human diaphragms were infected with trichinae. This is a significant reduction from the 16.1 percent prevalence found in similar studies conducted in 1931–42. Furthermore, the current study has shown that only 1.6 percent of individuals less than 44 years of age were positive compared to 4.6 percent for persons 45 years or older. (62)

Problems with Meat

The small larvae of the trichinae first get into the intestinal tract from the ingestion of infected meat. They can then migrate to the most active muscles of the body such as the calf muscle, the diaphragm, or the tongue. Rarely is the condition diagnosed even though aches and pains may occur. Cooking meat until the temperature in the center of the thickness of meat is 137° F. (58°C.) will destroy the larvae.

The trichinae originate in the hog. However, recent outbreaks are reported from the use of beef contaminated with the pork. In 1974, New Jersey had more cases of trichinosis from beef than from pork. One cause for this is that butchers, it seems, frequently avoid wasting pork scraps by throwing them in with beef. Also they use the same meat grinder for both pork and beef. The same knife is used to cut beef that is used to slice pork. It has been shown that trichinae may be transmitted on the knife. Regulations must be developed to require at least two meat grinders in each butcher's shop so that one will be used only for pork.

The large outbreak of trichinosis from beef in New Jersey alerted the entire nation to this problem. Further studies were done by the New Jersey health department and also by the National Center for Disease Control. It was found that as many as 8–20 percent of stores have beef contaminated with pork. (63, 62)

Meat Inspection

Meat inspection is of no value in the prevention of any of the disease hazards here discussed. Microscopic examinations are rarely made. When a cancer is found it is frequently removed and the remainder of the animal is sold for food. A knowledge of the spread of cancer within a body makes it evident that one who purchases such for food gets cancerous tissue.

Even though meat is stamped as safe because it has been inspected, 50 percent of it contains salmonellae, which makes it unsafe unless cooked properly. As most farmers know, sick animals are marketed if at all possible.

What is known about disease transmission in meat and meat products—and what is suspected but as yet unverified—renders meat a highly questionable food for use in a health-promoting diet.

Population Growth and Economics

The promotion of disease is far from being the only problem with meat as a food source. Its heavy drain on world energy and nutrition resources indicates the need for evaluating our traditional dependence on meat as a dietary staple.

With an increasing world population the use of animal food will have to be curtailed. Each second the earth's population increases by more than one person, each day by more than 100,000, and each year by more than 45 million persons (Ehrlich estimates 70 million). The present population will double in 35 to 40 years.

Problems with Meat

Energy Loss
in Use of Land
for Meat Production

LAND USE	FOOD PRODUCT	CALORIES
1 ACRE WHEAT	BREAD	800,000
1 ACRE GRAZING	MEAT	200,000
	ENERGY LOSS	600,000

Relative Efficiency
of Sources of Calories

Calories Used by Animal	Food Product	Calories Available from Food Product
100	MILK 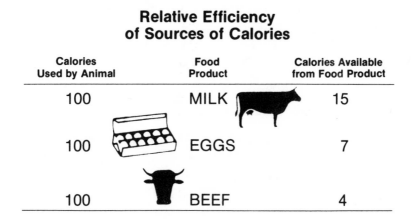	15
100	EGGS	7
100	BEEF	4

Problems with Meat

At the present rate of population growth, it has been estimated, quixotically perhaps, that the earth's surface will be completely covered with people in 700 years— and by 7,000 years from now people will have to go upwards, tier upon tier, at the speed of light. (8) Ridiculous? Probably. But it is a sobering fact that the population has already outgrown the food supply in many areas of the world, with resulting famine. By the year 2000 it is estimated there will be almost 6 billion, and by 2040, 12 billion people on earth—three times the present number. (8)

Greatest Source of Energy and Protein Loss

Land used to produce food crops for direct human consumption feeds 14 times as many people as land used to grow food for animals that are in turn used for human consumption. Plants will yield 800,000 calories per acre for direct human consumption, but only 200,000 when these same plant foods are first fed to animals. Thus meat animals use for themselves approximately 600,000, or three-fourths, of the calories from each acre's crop. Meat represents the greatest food energy loss in this country. Animals are obviously poor converters of calories for human consumption. Of the calories used by animals, only 15 percent are returned to humans in the form of milk, 7 percent as eggs, and 4 percent in the form of beef. (1, 57, 86)

Animals are also wasteful of protein itself. Of the protein that animals consume, only 23 percent is returned for human consumption in the form of milk, 12

Relative Efficiency
of Sources of Protein

Protein used by Animal, gm.	Food Product	Protein Available in Food Product, gm.
100	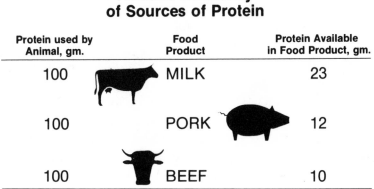 MILK	23
100	PORK	12
100	BEEF	10

Problems with Meat

percent in pork and 10 percent in the form of beef. Soybeans produce per acre 7.1 times more amino acids than cows in the form of milk and 8.2 times more than hens in the form of eggs when the land is used for animal feed. Soybeans will produce 17 pounds of protein per acre compared to 2 pounds for milk and 1 pound for beef.

Maximum Supportable Population

According to James Bonner, the maximum supportable world population is 50 billion, based on: (a) the total economy geared to food production, (b) cultivation of all land with the deserts being reclaimed by purified sea water (a major catastrophe such as a power breakdown could mean that 90 percent of the people would starve); and (c) the existence of no animals at all. (8)

Even a world food economy like that already existing in Japan would be like having the world populated with 16 billion people. This would be a very intensive food economy. If right now all of Asia had a food economy like that of Japan and the rest of the world like that of Western Europe, the world could support only 8–10 billion people. Even this would be attainable in 75–100 years only if agricultural production were to increase at 2 percent per year.

The Standard Nutrition Unit

A standard nutrition unit is defined as 2,500 calories per person per day. (1, 57, 86) A meat and milk diet requires three and one-half acres to supply one standard unit; a wheat and bread diet, one-fourth acre. A Japanese rice and bean diet will supply 6–7 units per acre. As population grows and food economy becomes a necessity, animal foods cannot be used.

Water is coming to be more in short supply. It takes energy to supply usable water and energy is also in short supply. Therefore, the cost of water is increasingly important. It takes 25 times more water to produce a pound of meat than it does to produce a pound of vegetables. For this reason alone meat must even now be de-emphasized as a source of human food in some parts of the world.

Cost of Foods Compared

A study we recently did for a television release by the Los Angeles County Medical Society demonstrated the economic advantage of a nonflesh diet, utilizing then prevailing prices.

Cost of Selected Foods Compared

	Cost 100 Calories	Cost 100 gm Protein	Cost Serving
Beans, kidney	3c	5c	3c/3 oz.
Potatoes, baked 15c/lb.	4c	15c	3c/3 oz.
Grains			
Oatmeal, cooked 30c/lb.	2c	5.1c	2.1c/ cup
Bread	3.2c	8.6c	2.1c/slice
Meats			
Hamburger, med.	8c	8c	18c/3 oz.
Wieners, pork	6c	11c	13c/3 oz.
Round steak	31c	18.5c	60c/3 oz.
Chicken, thigh	51c	22c	44c/3 oz.

Problems with Meat

Animal vs. Vegetable Protein
(per 100 Calories)

	ROUND STEAK		BEANS
Cost in cents		10.7	2
Calories		100	100
Protein, gm.		12.0	6
Carbohydrates, gm.		0.0	18
Fiber, gm.		0.0	1.3
Fat, gm.		5.5	.4

Also, in comparing the nutritional value of beans and steak it can be seen that beans are not only cheaper but even better nutritionally because they are so much lower in saturated fat.

Comparison of Animal vs. Vegetable Proteins

	Per 100 Grams		Per 100 Calories	
	Round Steak	Kidney Beans	Round Steak	Kidney Beans
Cost in cents	27.9	1.8	10.7	2
Calories	261	90	100	100
Grams	100	100	38	111
Protein, gms.	28.6	5.7	12.5	6.3
Calcium, mg.	130	40	4	44
Phosphorus, mg.	250	124	96	136
Iron, mg.	3.5	1.9	1.45	2.1
Vitamin A, I.U.	3	0	0	0
Vitamin B$_1$, mg.	0.08	0.05	0.03	0.05
Riboflavin, mg.	0.22	0.05	0.1	0.05
Niacin, mg.	5.6	0.8	2.35	0.9
Vitamin C, mg.	0	0	0	0
Fat, gm.	14.5	0.4	5.5	0.4
% Fat calories	47.3	3.4	47.3	3.4
P/S ratio	0.06	—	0.06	—
Carbohydrate, gm.	0	20	0	18

Problems with Meat

Some time ago the U.S. Department of Agriculture reported how much of the different nutrients you would get for a dollar spent on various food products. (85) (Although the prices of these foods have changed, their cost in relation to one another is still about the same.) A chart showing the amount of protein in a dollar's worth of various foods dramatizes the superior value of vegetable sources:

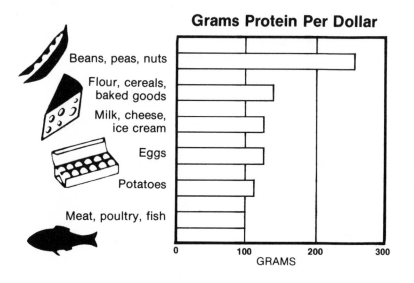

Grams Protein Per Dollar

Beans, peas, nuts

Flour, cereals, baked goods

Milk, cheese, ice cream

Eggs

Potatoes

Meat, poultry, fish

0   100   200   300
GRAMS

Problems with Meat

In a rating system devised by the author (see the "Best Buys" table), sugar and sweets are rated as the poorest buy—but next to them are meat and fish, not because there is not some good nutrition in meat but because it is proportionally very expensive.

In areas where people spend a large proportion of their income on food, the staples of diet are those foods in the four "highest value" categories listed in our table (cereals, legumes, potatoes, greens). Nutritionally and financially, such choices are a sound practice for everyone.

Best Food Buys

The "value points" assigned to these categories of foods reflect the frequency with which they appeared and their relative position in the U.S. Department of Agriculture tables of "best buy" sources of various nutrients. For a large number of nutrients, the six best buys were listed. Six points were assigned to the food group each time it rated first and so on, down to one point if rated only sixth as the most economical source of a nutrient. The "Best Food Buys" rating is a summary of the tables for all the nutrients.

$ Best Buys

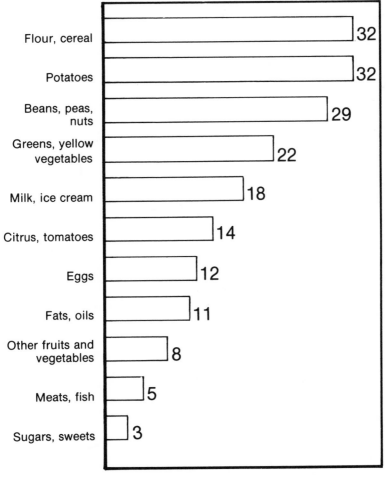

Flour, cereal	32
Potatoes	32
Beans, peas, nuts	29
Greens, yellow vegetables	22
Milk, ice cream	18
Citrus, tomatoes	14
Eggs	12
Fats, oils	11
Other fruits and vegetables	8
Meats, fish	5
Sugars, sweets	3

Based on Value Points Assigned by Author

Nutritional Problems of Meat

We often hear meat spoken of as some sort of "ideal" nutritional source that other kinds of foods must be measured by. Vegetable proteins are often spoken of as "possibly adequate"—if a great deal of thought and effort is applied to combining or otherwise using them to make them "almost as" nutritious as meat. This is nonsense—a result of many years of cultural conditioning.

The facts are: (1) A vegetable-based diet presents virtually no nutritional problems; (2) A meat-based diet presents complex, even grave, nutritional problems. Here are some of them.

Problems with Meat

Meat: A Carbohydrate-Deficient Food

Meat is a unique food in that it contains virtually no carbohydrates. While Americans are getting more than twice the amount of protein needed (55) and more than twice the amount of fat needed (18)—both of which contribute to serious disease problems—their diet is deficient in carbohydrates. An increase in carbohydrates in the American diet is one of the important goals of the Senate Select Committee on Nutrition and Human Needs. (78)

A lack of carbohydrates and an excess of either fat or protein is not conducive to either general well-being or physical endurance. Such popular diets as Stillman's or Dr. Atkin's, both high in protein and fat, have been shown to cause fatigue.

What is amazing is that the lack of endurance of meat eaters compared with vegetarians has been known and reportedly demonstrated for decades but it must continually be demonstrated anew. So engrained are traditional concepts about food!

Early in the 1920s the number of times vegetarians and nonvegetarians could squeeze a grip meter was compared. The vegetarians won with an average of 69 times; the nonvegetarians' average was only 38. Moreover, the vegetarians recovered from fatigue much more rapidly. (77). In another similar experiment, even the maximum record of the nonvegetarians was barely more than half that of the vegetarians. (27)

Recently a Swedish scientist gave nine athletes bicycle endurance tests after three-day periods on various

The Effect of Diet on Glycogen Stores and Physical Endurance

	Glycogen Content Per 100 g. Wet Muscle	Maximum Work Time
Normal Mixed Diet	1.75 gm.	114 minutes
Fat and Protein Diet (meats, fats, nuts)	.63 gm.	57 minutes
High Carbohydrate Diet	3.51 gm.	167 minutes

Problems with Meat

diets. (3) The diets were varied from high in meat (i.e., high in protein and fat) to high in vegetables and grains (i.e., high in carbohydrates). All the athletes were tested following periods on all of the diets so that differences in endurance could be accounted for only by differences in the diets.

When the athletes were on a high-fat and protein diet (high in meat content) their average endurance in the bicycle test was 57 minutes. After three days on the so-called normal mixed diet (lower meat, fat and protein) they averaged 114 minutes. On the high-carbohydrate diet (high in vegetables and grains) they averaged 167 minutes. Note that endurance was almost *three times greater* on the diet most resembling the vegetarian diet. This was accounted for, at least partly, by the higher and more sustained sugar (glycogen) content of muscle resulting from higher carbohydrate content of the diet.

High Fat Content of Meat

A major problem that has already been discussed is that the high fat content of meat is a major cause of both cancer and atherosclerosis. Also, concentrated forms of calories, as in meat, tend more readily to produce obesity. (89) Adult-onset diabetes occurs more commonly among the obese. Ironically, such diabetics formerly had been frequently placed on a meat-based, high-protein and fat diet. One result was increased mortality among diabetics due to atherosclerosis. Because we now know more about the hazards of high-protein, high-fat diets,

Health Hazards

Proportion of Decreased Life Expectancy Due to Atherosclerosis and Cancer Resulting From Various Causes

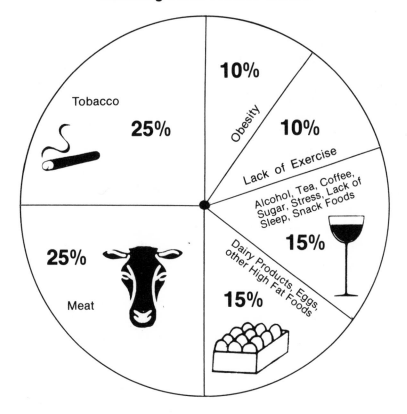

Tobacco

25%

10%

Obesity

10%

Lack of Exercise

Alcohol, Tea, Coffee, Sugar, Stress, Lack of Sleep, Snack Foods

15%

25%

Meat

Dairy Products, Eggs, other High Fat Foods

15%

Problems with Meat

present treatment for mild diabetes is primarily a high-carbohydrate diet. (16, 29) Such carbohydrates should be complex carbohydrates such as unrefined starches, rather than simple sugars, which are rapidly absorbed.

Excessive Protein in Meat

As has already been emphasized, Americans in general are getting twice as much protein as they need. (55) You will remember that high protein intake increases excretion of calcium (43, 52, 2)—tending to cause a loss of bone mass (osteoporosis) (2, 88, 24, 53)—increases the work of the liver and kidneys, (25, 82, 74, 76) and shortens life span. (80, 81, 46, 75, 25)

Surprisingly, high protein intake can also result in excessive vitamin losses. For example, because protein mobilizes vitamin A from the liver into the bloodstream, (73) high protein intake increases the requirement for Vitamin A and favors the onset of deficiency symptoms in animals. (73, 70) Such a diet also increases the requirement for Vitamin B_{12} or folate. (38, 22)

Thus, contrary to conventional "wisdom," it is the meat-based—not the vegetable-based—diet that presents the greater difficulties in obtaining adequate nutrition, that requires the more complex "computations" and careful "combinations."

Good Nutrition Is Difficult on a Meat Diet

There is great difficulty in teaching proper nutrition based on a meat diet. Here are some of the problems:

1. People must know the cholesterol content of animal foods so as not to exceed the recommended limit of 300 mg. per day. (42, 78)

2. A knowledge of the saturated fat content of various foods is necessary in order to observe the recommendation that such fat not exceed 10 percent of daily calorie intake. (42, 78)

3. If people need a therapeutic diet to lower their serum cholesterol (one-half the United States population has serum cholesterols above 210 mg. percent and should be on such a diet), they would have to be well informed regarding the saturated fat content of foods since in this case they would be allowed only 4 percent of their daily calories from fats. (58) They would need to know that a man on 2,700 calories daily could have no more than 12 grams of saturated fat a day. They would need to know that 3½ ounces of sirloin steak contain 13 grams of saturated fat and that the same amount of rib roast contains 16 grams.

4. Because it is important that carbohydrate intake be increased, it is a real problem for people on a meat diet to know how to increase their carbohydrate intake (without increasing calories) in order to be getting the Senate committee-recommended 55–60 percent of daily calories from carbohydrates (78). Actually, I recommend a diet with 70 percent of the calories from carbohydrates and only 20 percent from fat.

5. A similar problem appears in meat-based nutrition when we try to fulfill the need for more fiber, because meat contains none. With meat occupying a large part of the diet, people are hard pressed to know where they are

Problems with Meat

going to get enough fiber from the other foods in the diet. They must know the amount of fiber in various foods to ensure an adequate intake.

6. Because meat is low in calcium and increases the excretion of calcium, (43, 52, 2) a person on a meat diet must know how to ensure adequate intake of extra calcium to prevent osteoporosis, or loss of bone mass.

The reality of these problems is evident in the high mortality from cancer and atherosclerosis, among other disease problems, which makes it tragically obvious that it is not easy for the average person to learn how to eat properly on a meat diet.

In contrast, again contrary to conventional belief, it is simple for a vegetarian to maintain a healthful diet. There is no worry about cholesterol and little concern about saturated fat. Fiber and carbohydrate are adequate without any special calculation. How ironic that for so long it has been thought that it was the vegetarian who had difficulty in learning to get adequate nutrition!

Complete Protein Not Required at Every Meal

Wrong notions about the supposed difficulties and complexities of a vegetarian diet have arisen from an old idea—still believed even by many vegetarians—that it is necessary to have a proper mix of the essential amino acids, the chief components of protein, at every meal. (These are the amino acids the body cannot manufacture and that must therefore be derived directly from foods.)

Problems with Meat

Animal foods contain all the essential amino acids and their proportions are such that more of the absorbed protein is retained for body use than is the case with vegetable proteins. Therefore, when only one vegetable food was the whole diet, it has been thought that vegetable foods should be supplemented. The supplementation has been accomplished with milk or some animal protein or with a mixture of vegetable foods to increase the retention of the absorbed protein. It was thought that the biological value (the fraction of nitrogen of the protein source retained by the body) of plant foods should be equal to that of animal foods.

This old theory was based on studies between 1929 and 1950 using purified amino acids. (12, 31, 6) Rats fed half of the essential amino acids in one meal and half at subsequent meals had poor growth. (12) Other animals were fed all the essential amino acids with the exception of just one—either lysine or methionine. The missing amino acid, lysine or methionine, was fed to the animals 12 hours later in a protein-free meal. Again there was poor growth of the animals. (31, 6)

Studies of humans in which all the essential amino acids except tryptophan were fed demonstrated that the protein was of poor quality. The tryptophan had to be fed within one-half hour of the other amino acids in order to have a good quality protein. (6)

These observations led to the conclusion that a complete protein should be eaten at each meal. But remember these tests were conducted with purified amino acids. We don't eat pure amino acids. Only gelatin and protein isolates are completely devoid of one or more amino acids. Vegetable protein foods are not lacking totally in any specific amino acid.

New knowledge has completely reversed the old theory. In one experiment, dogs were fed either egg, zein (a deficient type of corn protein) or a completely protein-free diet. One and a half hours later a tube was placed in the intestines and the contents removed and analyzed for amino acids. From the analysis it could not be determined which dog had been fed which meal! It was concluded that enzymes from the intestinal juices helped to produce the missing amino acids. (59) Sloughed-off cells from the stomach probably also were a source of amino acids.

Other studies were done with rats. It was discovered that the protein of wheat (with a biological value that is limited by the amount of lysine it contains) is of the same quality whether lysine is added to it with the meal or given 4, 8, 12, or 16 hours after the meal. (91)

Again, animal studies were done on the biological value, growth factors, and protein efficiency ratios of wheat or zein products. When lysine was fed 12 hours after the meal, there was no important difference due to the time lag in giving the deficient amino acid. (6) These results occur, in contrast to the earlier purified amino acid studies, because foods are not lacking totally in any essential amino acid.

The conclusion is that it does not make any difference whether a complete protein is fed at each meal or not. There is no need to eat beans with grains, for example, to get the proper complementation of lysine and methionine. (In any case, growth rate—used for many

Problems with Meat

of these studies as a measure of protein value—may not be a good indicator of the ideal diet, because rapid growth frequently results in premature death!)

The old worries about a vegetarian diet being protein deficient are groundless and should be laid to rest. The truth is that protein is not lacking in any kind of usual diet in this country or in most countries of the world. It is actually difficult in this country to be protein deficient if one is getting calories adequate to maintain ideal weight.

Vegetable Sources of Protein

If you give up meat, milk, and eggs in order to lower serum cholesterol and to avoid other health hazards of animal foods, where will you get your protein? Especially if you are hypoglycemic and need more protein, where will it come from if you eliminate these high-protein foods from your diet? Cholesterol intake could be reduced by the use of nonfat milk and only the white of eggs—still providing plenty of animal protein. But how will those who wish to avoid even these animal products obtain adequate protein? These are common questions when one ventures into vegetarian ways.

But, as has been pointed out, these are for the most part not real problems. If you are maintaining your ideal

Problems with Meat

weight, whatever you are eating, you are likely, in a modern society, to be getting sufficient protein. Most foods contain protein even though they are not thought of as protein foods. Let me emphasize, it is difficult to design a reasonable experimental diet that provides an active adult with adequate calories that is deficient in protein.

If only 10 percent of the calories in an active adult man's diet of 2,700 calories (as recommended by the Food and Nutrition Board) were from protein, he would be getting more than enough protein to meet the Food and Nutrition Board's recommended allowance of 56 grams. If only 5 percent were from protein he would still meet the *minimum* requirement, with approximately 34 grams of protein.

Nitrogen loss each day is equivalent to approximately 20 grams of protein. In this case, if each day you took in 20 grams of protein of 100 percent biological value, you would meet your minimum protein requirement. If the biological value of the protein were only 60 percent, 33 grams of protein would be required. Most Americans have a diet with a protein biological value closer to 70 percent, which means that only 28 grams would be needed to maintain nitrogen balance.

How does this work out in a vegetarian diet? What percentage of the calories of common foods consist of protein? If one-third of the calories came from each of the following three groups, you would get 13 percent of your calories as protein—more than the recommended allowance.

⅓ Greens (30%)
Legumes (22%) 23%

⅓ Potatoes (8%)
Grains (7–14%) 8%

⅓ Fruits (8%)
Tomatoes (18%) 8%

Average of all calories as protein 13%

In practice, many vegetarians unfortunately "dilute" their calories with as much as 35 percent coming from visible fats and sugars. Even if you dilute your calories by 50 percent from such sources, you would still get 6½ percent of your calories as protein. Since 5 percent meets the *minimum* protein requirements, you would still be getting that even on an atrocious diet.

Lack of calories may cause a protein deficiency. Otherwise it is difficult to develop protein deficiency except in certain disease conditions.

A study of a small number of children in Guatemala that showed the intake of calories and protein compared to the recommended intake for ages 1 to 5. (87)

Calorie and Protein Intake
of Guatemalan Children
(as % of recommended intake)

	Years of Age			
	1	2	3	4-5
% Recommended Calories	63	66	80	48
% Recommended Protein	79	74	108	67

Problems with Meat

Although the three-year-olds got only 80 percent of the recommended calories, they obtained more than the recommended allowance of protein (108 percent). If calories were even close to adequate in the other age groups, the protein intake would be adequate.

Even in disease states such as kwashiorkor and marasmus, the problem is primarily a deficit of calories. In a few instances it is possible to demonstrate that even with enough calories there is a protein deficiency but this is rare. It may occur where a mother is feeding only starch because the child has diarrhea and the mother thinks this may soothe the intestinal tract. In Africa, where certain very low-protein roots are used heavily as staples, protein deficiencies may also be possible. (36)

In weight reduction, due to the limited caloric intake, some of the protein taken in is used for energy. Therefore, it may be useful to have a little more protein in such reducing diets. In this case, with the caloric intake low, the percentage of calories in the form of protein could be relatively high, if the absolute amount of protein taken in were the same.

For the hypoglycemic there are foods that are high in protein but not also high in saturated fats. For example, one could use nonfat milk, tofu or soybean curd (in many ways an excellent egg replacer); legumes such as beans, peas and lentils; "vegemeats" such as Vege-burger® (made from wheat gluten, soy flour and yeast) or soy-based "chicken"; brewer's yeast; wheat germ; or seeds such as sunflower or sesame seeds. Egg white contains the protein of the egg and could be used without the yolk to lower serum cholesterol. Nonfat cottage cheese could be used—and it can be tasty in loaves and other dishes.

Good Nutritional Status of Non-Meat Users

The nutritional status of non-meat users is good. They have greater life expectancy, (47) with approximately half the mortality from both coronary heart disease (67) and cancer, (48) compared with the general population.

Studies by Hardinge (35) on total vegetarians and lacto-ovo-vegetarians compared to nonvegetarians show adequate intakes of nutrients in all categories. The aver-

Problems with Meat

age intake of all groups approximated or exceeded the amounts recommended by the National Research Council's Food and Nutrition Board, with the exception of the adolescent total vegetarian—but even they obtained more than minimum requirements. No evidence was obtained to indicate that a lacto-ovo-vegetarian diet failed to provide adequate nutrition, even for pregnant women.

In general, height, weight, and blood pressure were similar in all groups except that the total vegetarian was 20 pounds lighter in weight. Serum total protein, albumin, globulin, and other blood chemistry findings were not statistically different.

The average vegetarian ingests adequate amounts of protein. (35) The amounts of essential amino acids in the diet not only meet the minimum requirements—they more than twice exceed them. (34)

For Your Reference:

A Rating
of Health Hazards

A Rating
of Health Hazards

When we rate the health hazards that decrease life expectancy from atherosclerosis and cancer, tobacco is the primary factor. Close behind it, however, is meat. Meat is high in fat, saturated fat, and cholesterol. Other high-fat foods of animal origin such as dairy products (cheese, butter, cream, ice cream) and eggs do their share in causing these diseases. Obesity and lack of exercise would be about equal as health hazards. Numerous other factors of lesser importance in atherosclerosis and cancer make up the balance of what I present here as "The Health Hazard Pole" (See graph.)

It has been shown that Seventh-day Adventist men have a 6.2-year greater life expectancy at age 35–40, half of which is due to not smoking. (47) The rest of the advantage is primarily due to using less meat. Adventist lacto-ovo-vegetarians have only two-thirds the coronary heart disease mortality, and Adventist total vegetarians only one-third the mortality of those Adventists who eat meat. (67) A high-animal fat diet increases the risk of heart attack and also of cancer of the colon, breast, and prostate. (90)

Obesity increases the risk of heart attack by increasing serum lipids, blood pressure and the incidence of diabetes. It also increases the risk in women of cancer of the uterus, kidney (90) and breast. (39) Moderate exercisers have only half as many heart attacks and one quarter as many deaths in the first 48 hours after the heart attack as those who are relatively inactive. (79)

A whole group of factors makes up the remainder of the hazards.

Note "Breslow's 7." Breslow has pointed out that observing only seven health habits can increase life expectancy by 11 years. (10, 4, 5)

Note also "Scharffenberg's 10." To Breslow's 7, I have added: saturated fats (meat, milk, hard fats); (9) stress (30) and sugar. (37, 78)

Problems with Meat

Notes on the "Health Hazard Pole"

A. *Tobacco*. Adventist men 35–40 years of age have 6.2 years' greater life expectancy. (47) Half of this is due to not smoking, (47) lessening incidence of heart attacks and cancer.

B. *Meat*. Almost half of the greater life expectancy of Adventist men is due to using less meat, which also lessens frequency of heart attacks and cancer.

C. *Dairy and Other High-Fat Foods*. Total vegetarians have only half the risk of coronary heart disease as lacto-ovo-vegetarians. (67) High-fat diet increases the risk of cancers of the colon, breast, and prostate. (90)

D. *Obesity*. Increases the risk of coronary heart disease and the risk in women of cancers of the uterus, kidney, breasts. (39)

E. *Lack of Exercise*. Moderate exercisers have half as many heart attacks and one-fourth as many fatalities in the first 48 hours following an attack as do inactive persons.

F. *Alcohol* . Decreases flow of blood through the heart, increases cancers of the esophagus, larynx, oral cavity. *Stress*. Increases the risk of coronary heart disease. (30)

The various hazards would change in relative position depending on the disease. For example, as a reducer of life expectancy from all causes, alcohol would be high on the list. In any case, these suggest major life-style changes needed in the American society and in other affluent societies today.

Health Hazard Pole

Decreased Life Expectancy from Atherosclerosis and Cancer

		Breslow's 7 (10, 4, 5)	Scharffenberg's 10 To Breslow's 7, add:
A	25% Tobacco	(Health habits. increase life expectancy by 11 years) 1. Tobacco	
B	25% Meat		8. Saturated fats (meat, milk, hard fats)
C	15% Dairy Products, Eggs, High-Fat Foods		
D	10% Obesity	2. Obesity	
E	10% Lack of Exercise	3. Exercise	
F	15% Alcohol, Tea, Coffee Stress, Sugar No Breakfast, Snacks Lack of Sleep, etc.	4. Alcohol 5. Breakfast 6. Snacks 7. Sleep	9. Stress (30) 10. Sugar (37, 78)

A Final Word

In the light of the formidable and persuasive scientific evidence we now have, let me simply summarize some major points that can dramatically affect your life.

Meat is an undesirable food because:
1. Meat is a major factor in of the leading causes of death in the United States, and probably in similar affluent societies. In fact, next to tobacco and alcohol, meat is the greatest single cause of mortality in the United States.
2. The cost of meat is excessively high.
3. Meat wastes energy when conservation is a necessity.
4. Meat is deficient in two major essential food components: carbohydrate and fiber.
5. It is difficult to plan and achieve good nutrition with a flesh diet.

The alternative diet, based on vegetarian principles, has none of these problems and promotes health and longevity.

For your own happiness, for your health, for your life—I encourage you to think about these facts and to use them in order to give yourself the greatest possible opportunity for an invigorating, long, and productive lifetime.

References

1. Altschul AM: Proteins, Their Chemistry and Politics. Basic Books, Inc., New York, 1965, pp. 262–65.
2. Anand CR, Linkswiler HM: Effect of protein intake on calcium balance of young men given 500 mg. calcium daily. J. Nutrition 104: 695–700, 1974.
3. Astrand P: Something old and something new. Nutrition Today 3: No. 2, 9–11, 1968.
4. Belloc NB: Relationship of health practices and mortality. Prev. Med. 2: 67–81, 1973.
5. Belloc NB, Breslow L: Relationship of physical health status and health practices. Prev. Med. 1: No. 3, 409–21, 1972.
6. Berg CP, Rose WC: J. Biol. Chemistry 82: 479, 1929.
7. Blankenship J (Loma Linda University): Personal communication.
8. Bonner J: The population dilemma. Bulletin (Los Angeles County Medical Society) 95: Jan. 21, 1965, pp. 9–12.

Problems with Meat

9. Boudreau FG: In Department of Agriculture: Food, The Yearbook of Agriculture, 1959, U.S. Government Printing Office, Washington, D.C., 1959, p. 16.
10. Breslow L: A quantitative approach to the World Health Organization definition of health. Int. J. Epidemiology 1: No. 4, 347–55, 1972.
11. Burkitt DP: Varicose veins, deep vein thrombosis, and haemorrhoids: Epidemiology and suggested aetiology. Br. Med. J. 2: 556–61, 1972.
12. Cannon PR, Steffee CH, Frazier LJ, Rowley DA, Stepto RC: The influence of time of ingestion of essential amino acids upon utilization in tissue-synthesis. Fed. Proc. 6: 390, 1947.
13. Carroll KK: Dietary factors in hormone-dependent cancers. In Winick M, ed.: Nutrition and Cancer. John Wiley and Sons, 1977, pp. 25–40.
14. Carroll KK: Experimental evidence of dietary factors and hormone-dependent cancers. Cancer Research 35: 3374–83, 1975.
15. Christakis G, Rinzler SH, Archer M, Kraus A: Effect of the anti-coronary club program on coronary heart disease risk-factor status. JAMA 198: 597–604, 1966.
16. Committee on Food and Nutrition, American Diabetes Association: Principles of nutrition and dietary recommendations for patients with diabetes mellitus: 1971. Diabetes 20: 633–34, 1971.
17. Committee on Nitrate Accumulation, National Academy of Sciences: Accumulation of Nitrate, National Academy of Sciences, 2101 Constitution Ave., Washington, D.C., 20418, 1972.
18. Conner WE, Conner SL: The key role of nutritional factors in prevention of coronary heart disease. Prev. Med. 1: 49–83, 1972.
19. Cummings JH: Progress report: Dietary fibre. Gut 14: 69–81, 1973.

20. Dayton S, Pearce ML, Hashimoto S, Dixon WJ, Tomiyasu U: A controlled clinical trial of a diet high in unsaturated fat in preventing complications of atherosclerosis. Circulation 40 (Suppl II): 1–63, 1969.
21. deGroot AP, Luyken R, Pikaar NA: Cholesterol-lowering effect of rolled oats. Lancet 2: 303–4, 1963.
22. Dryden LP, Hartman AM: Vitamin B_{12} deficiency in the rat fed high protein rations. J. Nutrition 101: 579–87, 1971.
23. Editor: Diet and stress in vascular disease. JAMA 176: 134–35, 1961.
24. Ellis FR, Holesh S, Ellis JW: Incidence of osteoporosis in vegetarians and omnivores. Am. J. Clin. Nutr. 25: 555–58, 1972.
25. Evans N: High protein ration as a cause of nephritis. California and Western Medicine, April, 1925, pp. 1–6.
26. Exton-Smith AN: Physiological aspects of aging: Relationship to nutrition. Amer. J. Clin. Nutr. 25: 853–59, 1972.
27. Fisher I: Yale Med. J., March 1907.
28. Food and Nutrition Board: Recommended dietary allowances, 1973, National Research Council, National Academy of Sciences, 2101 Constitution Ave., Washington D.C. 20418.
29. Friedman GJ: Diet in the treatment of diabetes mellitus. In Goodhart RS and Shils ME: Modern Nutrition in Health and Disease, Lea and Febiger, Philadelphia, 1973, pp. 846–47.
30. Friedman M, Rosenman RH: Association of specific overt behavior pattern with blood and cardiovascular findings. JAMA 169: 1286–96, 1959.
31. Geiger E, Hagerty EB: Importance of time factor upon utilization of amino acids in "maintenance" of adult rats. Fed. Proc. 9: 359, 1950.

Problems with Meat

32. Grace JT, Mirand EA, Mount DT: Relationship of viruses to malignant disease. A.M.A Arch. Int. Med. 105: 482–91, 1960.
33. Grace JT et al.: Canad. Cancer Conf. 4: 313–30, 1961.
34. Hardinge MG, Crooks H, Stare FJ: Nutritional studies of vegetarians. V. Proteins and essential amino acids. J. Am. Diet. Assoc. 48: 25–28, 1966.
35. Hardinge MG, Stare FJ: Nutritional studies of vegetarians. I. Nutritional, physical and laboratory studies. J. Clin. Nutr. 2: 73–82, 1954.
36. Hegsted DM: Deprivation syndrome or protein-calorie malnutrition. Nutr. Rev. 30: 51–54, 1972.
37. Hegsted DM: Priorities in nutrition in the United States. J. Am. Diet. Assoc. 71: 9–12, 1977.
38. Herbert V: The five possible causes of all nutrient deficiency: Illustrated by deficiencies of vitamin B12 and folic acid. Amer. J. Clin. Nutr. 26: 77–86, 1973.
39. Hirayama T: Paper presented at Conference on Breast Cancer and Diet, U.S.-Japan Cooperative Cancer Research Program, Fred Hutchinson Cancer Center, Seattle, Washington, March 14–15, 1977.
40. Huebner R: 70 newly recognized viruses in man. Public Health Reports 74: 6–12, 1959.
41. Interdepartmental Committee on Nutrition for National Defense: Manual for Nutrition Surveys, U.S. Government Printing Office, Washington, D.C. 20402, 1963, p. 250.
42. Inter-Society Commission for Heart Disease Resources. Report of Inter-Society Commission for Heart Disease Resources: Primary prevention of the atherosclerotic diseases. Circulation 42: A53–95, December 1970.
43. Johnson NE, Alcantara EN, Linkswiler H: Effect of level of protein intake on urinary and fecal calcium and calcium retention of young adult males. J. Nutrition 100: 1425, 1970.

44. Keys A, Grande F, Anderson JT: Fiber and pectin in diet and serum cholesterol concentration in man. Proc. Soc. Exp. Biol. Med. 106: 555–58, 1961.
45. Kralj-Cercek L: Human Biology 28(4): 393, 1956.
46. Krohn PL: Rapid growth, short life. JAMA 171: 461, 1959.
47. Lemon FR, Kuzma JW: A biologic cost of smoking. Arch. Environmental Health 18: 950–55, 1969.
48. Lemon FR, Walden RT: Death from respiratory disease among Seventh-day Adventist men. JAMA 198: 117–26, 1966.
49. Lijinsky W, Shubik P: Benzo(a)pyrene and other polynuclear hydrocarbons in charcoal-broiled meat. Science 145: 53–55, 1964.
50. Lutwak L: Current concepts of bone metabolism. Ann. of Int. Med. 80: 630–44, 1974.
51. Malmros H: The relation of nutrition to health. Acta Medica Scandinavia Suppl. No. 246, 1950.
52. Margen S, Chu JY, Kaufmann NA, Calloway DH: Studies in calcium metabolism. I. The calciuretic effect of dietary protein. Amer. J. Clin. Nutr. 27: 584–89, 1974.
53. Marsh AG, Keiser JA, Mayor GH, Mickelsen O, Sanchez TV: To fracture or not to fracture: clues that lacto-ovo-vegetarians offer us about protective health care. Abstract Book, Annual Meeting, American Dietetic Association, 1978, p. 74.
54. Mathur KS, Khan MA, Sherma RD: Hypocholesterolaemic effect of Bengal gram. A long-term study in man. Br. Med. J. 1: 30–31, 1968.
55. Mayer J (Harvard University): Family Health 5: 6 (Nov.), 1973.
56. Miettinene M, Turpeinen O, Karvonene MJ, Elosuo R, Paavilainene E: Effect of cholesterol-lowering diet on mortality from coronary heart-disease and other causes. Lancet 2: 835–38, 1972.

Problems with Meat

57. Morrison FB: Feeds and Feeding, The Morrison Publishing Co., Ithaca, N.Y., 1950, p. 261.
58. Mueller JF: A dietary approach to coronary artery disease. J. Am. Diet. Assoc. 62: 613–16, 1973.
59. Nasset ES: Role of the digestive tract in the utilization of protein and amino acids. JAMA 164: 172–77, 1957.
60. Nasset ES, Schwartz P, Weiss HV: The digestion of protein in vivo. J. Nutrition 56: 83–94, 1956.
61. National Academy of Sciences: An Evaluation of the Salmonella Problem. National Academy of Sciences, Washington, D.C., 1969.
62. National Communicable Disease Center: Trichinosis Surveillance. Annual Summary, 1968. National Communicable Disease Center, Atlanta, Georgia, May, 1969.
63. New Jersey State Health Department, Division of Environmental Health.
64. Nieman JM: The sensitizing carcinogenic effect of small doses of carcinogen. Europ. J. Cancer 4: 537–43, 1968.
65. Phillips RL (Loma Linda University): Personal communication, research report in press.
66. Phillips RL: Role of life-style and dietary habits in risk of cancer among Seventh-day Adventists. Cancer Research 35: 3513–22, 1975.
67. Phillips RL, Lemon FR, Hammond C: Coronary heart disease mortality among Seventh-day Adventists with differing dietary habits. Abstract American Public Health Association meeting, Chicago, Ill., November 16–20, 1975.
68. Phillips RL, Lemon FR, Beeson WL, Kuzma JW: Coronary heart disease mortality among Seventh-day Adventists with differing dietary habits: a preliminary report. Am. J. Clin. Nutr. 31: S–191–S–198, 1978.
69. Phillips RL, Lemon FR, Beeson WL, Kuzma JW: The Adventist Health Study, Educational Materials Center, School of Health, Loma Linda University, Loma Linda, CA.

70. Rechcigl M, Jr., Berger S, Loosli JK, Williams HH: Dietary protein and utilization of vitamin A. J. Nutrition 76: 435–40, 1962.
71. Reddy BS, Wynder EL: Large bowel carcinogenesis: fecal constituents of populations with diverse incidence rates of colon cancer. J. Natl. Cancer Inst. 50: 1437–42, 1973.
72. Rigdon RH, Neal J, Mack J: Leukemia in mice fed benzo(a)pyrene. Tex. Rep. Biol. Med. 25: 553–57, 1967.
73. Roels OA: Vitamin A physiology. JAMA 214: 1097, 1967.
74. Ross MH: Nutrition, disease and length of life. Ciba Foundation Study Group No. 17, Diet and Bodily Constitution. Little, Brown and Co., Boston, 1964, pp. 90–103.
75. Ross MH: Protein, calories and life expectancy. Fed. Proc. 18: 1190–1207, 1959.
76. Ross MH, Batt WG: Diet-age pattern for hepatic enzyme activity. J. Nutrition 61: 39, 1957.
77. Schouteden A: Ann. de Soc. Des Sciences Med. et Nat. de Bruxelles (Belgium) I. 1924.
78. Senate Select Committee on Nutrition and Human Needs: Dietary Goals for the United States. U.S. Government Printing Office, Washington, D.C., 20402, 1977.
79. Shapiro S, Weinblatt E, Frank CW, Sager RV: Incidence of coronary heart disease in a population insured for medical care (HIP). Am. J. Public Health 59 (Suppl.):1–101, 1969.
80. Sherman HC: Chemistry of Food and Nutrition, The MacMillan Co., New York, 1952, p. 208.
81. Sherman HC: The Science of Nutrition, Columbia University Press, New York, 1943, pp. 177–98.
82. Shilling E: Nutr. Abstr. & Rev. 33: 114, 1963.
83. Shimkin MB, ed. : Ca—A Cancer Journal for Clinicians 24: No. 3, 189, 1974.

84. Strom A, Jensen RA: Mortality from circulatory diseases in Norway 1940–1945. Lancet 1: 126–29, 1951.
85. U.S. Department of Agriculture, Agriculture Research Service: Family Food Plans and Food Costs, Home Economics Research Report No. 20, 1962, U.S. Department of Agriculture, Washington, D.C.
86. U.S. Department of Agriculture: Protecting Our Food, Yearbook of Agriculture, 1966, U.S. Government Printing Office, Washington, D.C., 1966, p. 359.
87. Viteri FE, Arroyave G: Protein-calorie malnutrition. In Goodhart S, Shils ME: Modern Nutrition in Health and Disease, Lea and Febiger, Philadelphia, 1973, p. 607. Table modified from : Flores, M et al.: Arch. Latino-Amer. Nutr. 20: 41, 1970.
88. Wachman, A, Bernstein DS: Diet and osteoporosis. Lancet 1: 958–59, 1968.
89. Wooley OW: Long-term food regulation in the obese and nonobese. Psychosomatic Medicine 33: 436–44, 1971.
90. Wynder EL: The dietary environment and cancer. J. Am. Diet. Assoc. 71: 385–92, 1977.
91. Yang SP, Clark HE, Vail GE: Effects of varied levels and a single daily supplement of lysine on the nutritional improvement of wheat flour proteins. J. Nutrition 75: 241–46, 1961.
92. Yang SP, Steinhauer JE, Masterson JE: Utilization of a delayed lysine supplementation. J. Nutrition 79: 257–61, 1963.
93. Allen LH, Oddoye EA, Margen S: Protein-induced hypercazciuria: a longer term study. Am. J. Clin. Nutr. 32:741-49, 1979.